Labor and Delivery in Rhyme

By Alpha

Too many years ago, I attended Jefferson Medical College and during one of our lectures we were introduced to The Acute Abdomen in Rhyme, written by Zeta. It is suspected that Zeta was really Sir Zachary Cope, author of Cope's Early Diagnosis of the Acute Abdomen. Although this text was somewhat simplistic, it was an excellent starting point for a medical student both in understanding the pathological processes behind and the diagnosis of conditions such as acute appendicitis, cholecystistis, bowel obstruction and a variety of other conditions that cause abdominal pain.

In The Acute Abdomen in Rhyme, Zeta wrote:

"The use of rhyme in teaching is quite small,

It's limitations great and plain to all

But use it has, although it may be merely

To put some things more quaintly or more clearly...

Well, wait and see, at least this I can state

A rhymster needs to think and concentrate,

And choose his words more carefully than those

Who oft repeat themselves in common prose....

My aim, which well may be I shall not reach,

Is to amuse you while I try and teach."

This is my attempt to do the same in Obstetrics. If I have failed to amuse you, at least I have succeeded in amusing myself.

Alpha

3

For BetaBeauty, my true love…………..

Table of Contents

Evaluation of the Patient in Labor

Mrs. Smythe will call you on the phone

And tell you she believes she should leave home.

While you listen she presents her case.

Her contractions previously were spaced,

But now are coming twelve within an hour

And when they peak her face is looking dour.

Into L&D she now will head.

It's the kind of phone call that you dread.

At two am you leave your comfy bed.

In place of sleep you know its work instead.

Now you could lie back down and fall asleep

And wait for your drat pager to go "Beep"

But with her second baby there's a chance

She might arrive in labor quite advanced.

And ne'er before you even don your pants

She will be delivered by Nurse Vance.

So into the big hospital you drive

Eyes a'squinty, feeling half alive.

The elevator to the eighth you take

The smile you give the Smythes is very fake.

But young OB's let me make this clear.

Nine tenths of L&D is being there.

Once arrived the patient you assess.

It's tempting to take shortcuts I confess.

But doing so can leave you quite a mess.

'Tis better to do more instead of less.

First, peruse the record, look to see

That there is an exacting EDC.

Prenatally, were there complications?

Medical conditions, exacerbations?

Laboratory tests and ultrasounds.

Group B strep cultures must be found.

Armed with information from the chart

You now can listen to the lungs and heart

Without the fear that the Smythes will mention

A problem that requires your attention

About which you know not a thing at all

You stammer and you blush and hem and haw

To late to now go running for the chart

Which you should have studied from the start.

As the physical exam unfolds

Including those maneuvers Leopold.

Try to be as thorough as you can

Instead of a derisory exam.

Reflexes, blood pressure and edema

Is that gestationis or eczema?

Are there lesions on the perineum?

If you don't look you'll surely never see 'em

While rushing to check cervical dilation,

Effacement, presentation and the station.

If the presenting part you cannot reach

Make certain it's a vertex not a breech.

In fact, even when the head is quickly found

There's information gleaned from ultrasound.

Although an extra penny you won't earn

By doing scans, this is how we learn.

With Mrs. Smythe in labor that is active

Accompanied by a tracing that's reactive.

Now the nurse will do you a great favor

Watching like a hawk while Ms. Smythe labors.

You must stay close and always heed her call.

'Tis no low risk in labor, none at all.

Uteri can rupture, cords can fall.

Blood pressure can rise, watch for it all.

Expect the unexpected, be prepared

Lest the night turn into a nightmare.

The Birth Plan

On the Internet, one can find

A list of things to keep in mind

When coming in to have a baby.

'I need these things, Doc. Don't say 'maybe'."

"I'd like to labor in a tub

My doula there my back can rub

And we can skip the intravenous

That Dr. Bradley calls so heinous

It leads to medical intervention

And other acts of pure convention

That certainly are not for us.

Oh, we don't want to make a fuss

But need you to respect our wishes

"What! Water births are just for fishes?"

And to prevent a lot of strife

We think a midwife would be nice

Of course, doc, you should be there too

If complications do ensue

She'll call you quick, right on the double

And you can get us out of trouble

But we expect things to go smooth

In which case, don't get in our groove.

That monitor will tie me down

And fill the room with dreadful sound.

We might not hear the string quartet

Playing in our tape cassette.

It's good to have an open mind

But with experience one will find

That all the strange things on the list

These things on which she doth insist.

Go quickly flying from the brain

When she confronts that labor pain.

Her husband, who invoked discussion

Lies on the floor with a concussion

And after several primal screams

She joins the epidural queens.

Thus, all these lists of man and wife

Falter in view of this thing called life.

And Fate perched high above in Heaven

Scoffs when he gets to number seven.

The head gets stuck, she won't dilate

We wait and wait and wait and wait.

And despite the careful plans they made

She's birthed with a shiny Bard Parker blade.

Management of the Patient in Labor

A wise Doc gave this sage advice:

Never let the sun set twice

Upon a woman laboring.

In this regard we're favoring,

As opposed to "wait and see,"

A style that dictates actively

Looking at all the important five P's.

Carter once admonished me:

"Before you cut you better see

That her contractions are up to snuff.

She's on some Pit, is it enough?"

Maybe an intrauterine tranducer

Should be used when you induce her.

A catheter inside the womb

Helps you decide there isn't room

With no descent and no dilation

The vertex stays at a high station

She is contracting adequately

Then you can call it CPD

Unless the baby is OP

Which is a common malady.

But either way, you can be sure

The kid's not coming out that door

And make a well thought out decision

To birth the child with an incision.

The first P for a vaginal birth

Is assessment of the Pelvic girth

Bones come in various shapes and sizes

A good obstetrician always apprises

If gynecoid or anthropoid apply

Since platypoid and android oft deny

Access to that bony pelvic bowl

And thwart vaginal delivery as a whole.

Next the Passenger's size one should assess

Though this may be in error I confess

Even when done by ultrasound

The weight may be mistaken by a pound.

The Powers that push the baby out

Are the next thing to think about.

One can judge contractions externally

But only in so far as frequency.

To calculate Montevideo units

The uterus needs a sensor in it.

Long ago Friedman had the verve

To put on graph a normal labor curve.

More recently others have inferred

That when he did his grid he might have erred.

Six centimeter now's considered active

So though Cesarean might seem attractive

Another P called Patience would be great

To help reduce your high C-section rate.

In this regard the P that's called Provider

Is well known to the L&D insider.

The nurses there all know just who you are

The doctor who decides to make a scar

To get there for a kid's big football match

Or so eight hours sleep, she's sure to catch.

So please don't be so quick to grab the knife

To get to early dinner with your wife.

You may think that you've won them with your charm.

But they all know you're doing patients harm.

And 'though you are the best Doc in the land

When you are home in bed you're not so grand.

Medications in Labor and Delivery

During the standard six week rotation

Medical students have the occasion

To master the drugs on L&D

Because, within our specialty,

Unlike in the ICU,

The drugs in L&D are few.

And so without delay or undue fuss

The drugs of L&D we'll now discuss.

Oxytocin

In the posterior pituitary there resides

Oxytocin, a small but important peptide.

(It's not alone, it lives in sin

Cohabitating with vasopressin)

Scientists have synthesized it

We call it Pitocin, or for short, Pit.

These nine amazing amino acids

Prevent a lazy uterus from being flaccid.

For a moment here, let me digress.

When laboring patients fail to progress

The quality of contractions we must assess

And if those contractions are hypotonic

Rather than wait, we should get right on it

For augmenting labor it's Pit we use.

Carefully watching how much we infuse.

(The dose is measured in mIU's.)

Too much will cause contractions tetanic

And throw the OB into a panic

If the uterus we hyperstimulate

Its sometimes reflected in the fetal heart rate.

The decelerations that were caused

Will disappear when the infusion is paused.

'Though braver souls will halve the rate

Rather than the entire infusion to negate.

This works as well experts report

Since the half-life of Pit is very short.

Oxytocin also is commonly prescribed

After the placenta has arrived

Here the dose is larger indeed

We don't want the uterus to bleed

So tetanic contraction is what we need.

Constricting the vessels in the decidual plate

After a while we can decrease the rate

But if the bleeding begins again

A constant infusion we'll have to maintain.

Methergine

Another drug that is commonly seen

On L&D is called Methyergonovine

By those whose like to speak generic.

Methergine is the brand name Erich.

This semi-synthetic ergot alkaloid

For uterine atony is also employed.

The dose is point two milligrams (0.2)

Whether given by mouth or given IM.

On the uterine muscle there is direct action

Producing sustained tetanic contraction.

But one must be aware of the contraindication.

Do not use Methergine when there is hypertension.

Hemabate

This drug is one we use for bleeding

When blood is flowing and sweat is beading

Despite the rapid Pitocin drip

And a shot of Methergine in the hip

At those times one dare not pause

The steady uterine massage.

And while the doctor has her hand in

She'll yell, "Nurse, get some prostaglandin.

On the double, don't make me wait.

We need an amp of Hemabate!

Carboprost tromethamine

Is badly needed at this scene!"

To help treat uterine atony

When it has been refractory

To other therapeutic modalities.

It helps prevent fatalities.

Terbutaline

Sometimes contractions can be good

Other times we wish they would

Go away, that is, abate

So the cervix does not dilate.

Mag sulfate for this is often used

But we might want a med that doesn't infuse.

And instead of using Nifedipine

We sometimes choose Terbulatine

This Beta 2 drug has a rapid action

Of inhibiting uterine contraction.

It's also used for cephalic version

And in cases of uterine inversion.

It makes the uterus a flaccid sac

Which aids in putting the fundus back.

And lets us turn the babe around

So the head points at the ground.

Also, with uterine tachysystole

Terbutaline can be given IV.

Misoprostol

Somehow they did not suspect

When manufacturing Cytotec

That misoprostol would come to be

A way to end maternity.

Still, as an agent for induction

Cytotec aids reproduction

And also works when we have the need

To treat a vexing postpartum bleed.

Betamethasone

Graham Liggins and Little Bo Peep

Concerned themselves with wooly sheep.

Bo wanted to get them home.

Graham gave Betamethasone.

Which did not do as he intended.

Preterm birth was never ended.

But the lambs had this salvation:

Accelerated lung maturation.

And thus in 1972

A research paper did ensue

Liggins and his friend Ross Howie

Made the Ob world say, "Wowie"

Their antenatal steroid trial

(A paper that I keep on file.)

Showed steroids give to babes this blessing

Much less chance of RDSing.

Their lungs surfactant will produce

It's this that steroids will induce.

(It also helps them to refrain

From bleeding in their tiny brain.)

Now when we reach week thirty-four

We don't use steroids anymore.

For patients seen before this time

Keep Betamethasone in mind.

With preterm labor it is clear

A preterm infant might appear.

But often with other conditions

We aren't quite as good clinicians

We can forget, I must confess

To treat the gal with PES

Or those that show up with a bleed

If early, steroids too they need.

Likewise, if their waters break.

Don't forget for goodness sake.

Antihypertensives

For some it comes as a surprise

When blood pressure begins to rise

And if they thereby hesitate

Intervention may come too late.

Cerebral autoregulation

May fail due to procrastination

Unfortunately this may lead

To an intracranial bleed.

Hydralazine or Labetolol

Simply stated, should be given to all

Patients who manifest severe hypertension

Because it is only by this intervention

That we prevent the tragedy

Of a maternal fatality.

Systolics 160! Sake's alive!

Or diastolics 105!

Give Labetolol! Don't even blink!

Believe me, you don't have to think.

Bells should be ringing, you should hear an alarm.

Giving 20 mg will do no harm.

The harm is in failing to act

Or denying the pressure, when in fact

The blood pressure continues to spike

And doesn't come down as you would like.

Magnesium Sulfate

In an English town called Surrey,

To which the afflicted with dropsy would scurry,

Flows the precious Epson spring.

To which many their loves would bring

Hoping to find an earthly Elysium

By bathing in waters with Sulphate of Magnesium

In 1910, was Ballantyne

Who somehow had the strength of mind

To take the waters of Epson Lake

And with saline an infusion make.

Which he administered IV

To eclamptics who were seizing you see

Nine patients did he treat this way

In doing so held death at bay.

I'm sure some thought that he was lying

When he cured them all with not one dying.

But the Brits chose to ignore

Their own magnesium sulfate lore.

Lazard in America in '25.

Used Mag to keep eclamptics alive.

Then Stroganov and Davidovitch

In Russia got the Mag sulfate itch.

Later there was some confusion

About giving Mag sulfate by infusion

'Cause Prichard at that Parkland place,

A doctor concerned with saving face.

Told his boys if you worked for him

You could only give the Mag IM.

Later, in 1978.

Zuspan again set us straight.

Treating patients at the Lying In,

In Chicago, gave Mag IV again.

Then began the big debate.

Dilantin better? Or Mag sulfate?

'Cause the chaps across the pond

Of Phenytoin were very fond.

The Collaborative Eclampsia test

In 1995 put this issue to rest.

The Yanks were certainly cheerier

When Mag was proved superior.

Mag works as a tocolytic

And a potent diuretic

And gives neuroprotection too

To babes that come before they're due.

All these gifts, from just one med

From a natural spring and the lake it fed.

The next time you are feeling smart

When treating ills from hip to heart

Ask why we cannot create

A medication that is as great

'Tis a miracle that God would bring

Those healing waters from Epson Spring

I know there is a bigger plan

That dwarfs the vanities of man.

Nifedipine

For some it came as quite a shocker

That this calcium channel blocker

Could be used to stop contractions

Now it's clear it has this action.

As a first line tocolytic

Procardia has many critics

And for maintenance tocolysis

There is no evidentiary basis.

Nifedipine is most renowned

For bringing high blood pressure down.

And what here is the most engrossing

Is an option for daily dosing.

Hypertension one can quell

Using Procardia XL.

Fetal Monitoring

In '70 there were first seen

Commercial EFM machines

Spawned by Drs. Hon and Paul

They held the Labor men in awe.

With hopes and dreams they were infused

Wanting that they could be used

To save from an uncertain fate

The life of any neonate.

Before this, still it was well known

And with outcomes easily shown

That the fetal heart rate dropped

When oxygen to the fetus stopped.

But to note the fetal rate

The nurses had to auscultate.

Alas, 'though the fetal heart was checked

For newborn lives there was neglect

In past times, Cesarean section

Was complicated by infection,

Hemorrhage and risk of aspiration.

Imagine one's exasperation

In knowing for Mom to survive

The baby won't be born alive.

Of course today, we intervene

When ominous tracings are seen

The most recent chapter in this story

Involves the use of category.

With moderate variability and no deceleration

Category one is the designation.

Bad tracings have come to be

Designated Category three.

With Three and One clinical decision

Does not require erudition

But most tracings are Category Two

And here's where we get in a stew.

OB experts can't agree

When viewing retrospectively

Strips with both good and bad features.

Some are also fickle creatures.

And to their own words will turn traitor

When they review strips six months later.

Plus, using hindsight, it's not fair

To pillory those providing care

Knowing outcomes is shown to sway

Opinions on a given day.

The recent terminology

Is better for psychology

Terms like tachysystole

Do not emote an injury

Likewise, Category two

Means naught unless defined for you.

I think it's much better to use

Terms that laymen might bemuse

Not those with an affective component

That aids the smarmy plaintiff's proponent.

The trial attorney's heart is racing

If heard: "Non reassuring fetal heart rate tracing."

The terms "severe" and "hyperstimulation"

Induce in him a palpitation.

And if he reads "fetal distress"

His underwear becomes a mess.

Like so many human schemes

EFM didn't meet our dreams

It didn't stop cerebral palsies

Because most often, we don't cause these

The EFM can just record

It can't predict a prolapsed cord

Nor help shoulders get unstuck

Or make up for the bad luck

Of a 3 a.m. abruption

Or a vasa previa's eruption.

Obstetrical emergency

Is something no one can foresee.

For labor there is this preamble:

You can't have gain without some gamble.

So why do patient's think that we

Should be on par with deity?

Preterm Labor and Delivery

Unfortunately, it oft' ensues

That babies come before they're due

And there is more than just one reason

That they are birthed in the wrong season.

Some Mom's sport a bad collection

Of intrauterine infection.

Others sprout a fluid leak

Before the thirty-seventh week.

Abruption also has the action

Of causing uterine contraction.

Twins and multiple gestation

Uterine cavity bifurcation

And cervical incompetence

May cause labor to commence.

But most often we don't know why

They're born before they're fit to cry.

There are some tests that can portend

A pregnancy's untimely end.

With second trimester ultrasound

A shortened cervix might be found

fFN might be used to pick

Between real labor and Brackton Hick.

But is there anything we can do

To keep the babe from the ICU?

Yes, steroids help the lungs mature
This we certainly know for sure.
But when it comes to stopping labor
Drugs work then fall into disfavor.

We once used ethyl alcohol
But then it didn't work at all
Magnesium, then terbutaline
FDA approved Ritodrine
Nifedipine and indocin
And now Mag is in vogue again.
They all might work to stop contraction
But do they really have the action
Of stopping labor when it's real?
Or is this just some misplaced zeal?

To know if we are doing harm
We'd need a matched placebo arm
And what mother should be entreated
To be the one who isn't treated.
Then by the time the study's done
Another decade has begun
Oh, and did I fail to mention
We still think in three dimensions.

Preeclampsia

You'd think that in this scientific age

There would arise some brilliant doctor sage

Who would the cause for PES make clear.

But, for now the question still is here.

No Noble Prize; no genius Doc to thank.

The plaque at Lying In remains a blank.

And no one yet can tell us why.

Mom's get sick and sometimes die.

Those who want a claim to fame

Seem to always change the name.

So much it seems, that I fear

The name will soon change twice a year.

Toxemia then. Now PES.

A better term, I must confess.

But, alas, such literary invention

Provides not cause or prevention.

Classically, blood pressure starts to rise.

Edema may be pitting to the thighs.

Protein in the urine may start to spill

Without the patient even feeling ill.

And in fact she may be astonished

Or not accept treatment, and be admonished

To comply with the treatment regimen

And the series of lab tests that will begin.

CBC with platelets and a urine screen

For urine protein and creatinine.

Tests to measure the function of the liver.

While we ask the question, "Do we deliver?"

To answer that question, as a start

Make a graph, a kind of chart

Time on one axis, Death on the other

To spare the baby, you risk the mother.

Thus, when there is severe disease

One should feel quite ill at ease.

And with HELLP syndrome, Jackson would shout,

"You better get the baby out!"

'Tis truly a dilemma when the baby is preterm

Oh, what a sharpened screw whose turning makes us
squirm.

One gives the patient steroids, the lungs one must mature.

Magnesium sulfate, the patient must endure.

It's a narrow tightrope on which the perinates must balance

Giving both eclampsia and prematurity their allowance.

Here's the art in medicine, to make that tough decision

When is it time for that Cesarean incision?

It's a sad day, when the baby is dead.

But sadder still, if you lose mother instead.

However, still there are Docs that think

They can take mother, right to the brink.

Giving medication to drop the pressure down,

Following their Doppler's with their ultrasound.

Pontificating, feeling smug as a bug

Until preeclampsia pulls out the rug.

Why were they waiting for the platelets to drop,

For that intracranial bleed, for the liver to pop,

For DIC, from that 4 a.m. abruption,

Or ARDS, with a prolonged induction.

Ninety nine times of course they are right.

But that one case will keep them sleepless at night.

After delivery, we still can't be sure

Although most times, delivery is the cure.

Some presentations, will be very atypical

Going by rote, may prove inimical.

Some will need magnesium, for more than 24 hours.

Be confined to bed and kept out of the shower.

Seizures can occur even after several days

Beware, postpartum headache, this syndrome has its ways

Of making one look silly and certainly misled,

When their "stable" patient, is thrashing on the bed.

Remember it's a syndrome and it doesn't follow rules

It hasn't read the textbook and it doesn't suffer fools.

There's still a lot to learn, about this strange condition

So don't preach me the gospel, while you're citing your edition.

Postpartum Hemorrhage

The baby lies against the mother's chest

Tempting now to let your mind just rest

But before this luxury you savor

Best to tend to the third stage of labor.

Why is it some patients have the need

To spoil the moment with a massive bleed

Or retain the placenta when it's due

"Placenta, here's the baby! Where are you!"

Sometimes the resident basks in glory

Unaware that there's more to the story

Than getting the baby from the womb

To the safety of the labor room.

All advice is now ignored

As he puts traction on the cord.

Under the gloves, we break a sweat

Hoping that we won't regret

Not taking over for that lout

So the uterus doesn't turn, inside out.

And what's this action with the fist?

Perhaps he hasn't got the gist

Of preventing a uterine inversion.

Who started this third stage perversion?

'Cause unless one isn't really dumb

They'll hold the womb up with their thumb

With fingers at the fundal top,

Feel a V? You'd better stop.

There is a constant third stage debate

Whether to give oxytocin early or late.

Me? I like to give Pit before

The placenta falls out toward the floor.

When the placenta takes its time

Another thing to keep in mind

Are anomalies of the decidual plate

So before you excavate

Consider Accreta and her sisters

Or else you'll be doing emergency hysters.

These are better done in a controlled fashion

Without the hemorrhage and all that splashin'.

When uterine atony causes this mess

Of postpartum hemorrhage, make sure you compress

The uterus, no need to be rough,

But fundal massage is not enough.

It should be bimanual with elevation

And done without much hesitation.

While you give your IV Pit,

And all those other meds with it,

Like Methergine and Hemabate

And Cytotec, for which we wait.

While down the hall the nurse goes zoom

'Cause they're no longer in the room.

Sometimes hemorrhage is colossal indeed

And with these cases there is the need

To summon help, all hands on deck

Get to the OR, where you can check

Everything that might be bleeding.

Granted the patient might be needing

O'Leary, B-Lynch or the Bakri balloon

But sometimes they're employed too soon.

Cervical or vaginal laceration

May be the source of exsanguination.

The OR has the advantage too

That anesthesia can watch the patient for you.

And also don't forget to call

For the massive transfusion protocol.

Finally, some patients need

Extended Pit so they don't bleed

For if the uterus fills with clot

It won't contract and they'll bleed a lot

By now the epidural's out

You check them and they thrash and shout

And again you hear them scream

Because you called the IV team

You could have saved them all this pain

With oxytocin in their vein.

Here it's important to remember, for sure

An ounce of prevention betters liters of cure.

Abruption

Functioning as both the lung and liver,

The placenta, that amazing life giver,

Forms villi that float in venous lakes.

It's also the form the attachment takes

Connecting the baby to the mother.

But there's a problem like no other

When the vessels in the spongiosum

Start to bleed and then let go some.

Usually the decidual plate

Doesn't start to separate

Before a living child is born.

But if the afterbirth is shorn

Before the birth there is disruption

Known as a placental abruption

And bleeding can be very great.

The bleeding will itself create

Uterine irritability and contraction

Which, by nature, has the action

Of causing more to separate

And this may seal the baby's fate.

A wise clinician is sure to heed

Any complaint regarding a bleed

Especially after the 23rd week.

Advise the patient to rapidly seek

Care on the labor and delivery floor

For this is the only way to be sure

The bleed is not an early sign of something more.

The health of mom and baby you must insure.

Though bleeding is usually the cardinal sign

There are other symptoms to keep in mind.

The blood may flow, or may by chance

Not end up in the patient's pants.

Occult abruption forms a retroplacental collection

Which may progress in a different direction.

And rather than a membranous dissection

The myometrium is its predilection.

So with pain but no bleeding, still beware

Lest you fail to note a Couvelaire.

Some patients are more at risk

For the placenta to dehisce

Those with uncontrolled hypertension

Or with uterine distension

As is seen in twin gestations

Or polyhydramnios, which has a relation.

As do women with high parity

And those who lack the clarity

To throw away their cigarettes

Or who use crack cocaine without regrets.

Thrombophilics abruptions see

As do those with high AFP's.

Also those who imbibe alcohol

(The proper amount is none at all.)

One cause to be mentioned in particular

Is trauma such as accidents vehicular.

Seatbelts should be worn of course

Still, deceleration causes a shearing force.

Be wary lest the novice be misled

By the patient resting quietly in bed.

There is no pain and she has yet to bleed.

But to those small contractions please take heed.

The signs and symptoms may be very subtle.

Ignoring them will get you into trouble.

A small abruption often will resolve

But, other times continues to evolve

Grade 1 becomes Grade 2 and then Grade 3.

There is no place for complacency

Or sending OB trauma out the door

Without being very, very sure

That of the uterine placentation

There has not been untimely separation.

Management decisions can be made

By classifying abruption by grade.

Grade 1 is called a Herald bleed

With blood loss less than 100 cc.

Marginal sinus separation

Falls into this classification

Treatment is for most part passive

Fetal heart rate is reactive

And the patient's fibrinogen

Which may have dropped will rise again.

So after days of observation

Which does require hospitalization

The patient's symptoms stay at bay

And if her term is far away

She may go home, not disregarded

For fetal growth may be retarded

Placenta infarcts might be found

So monitoring and ultrasound

Are used, providing a solution

To assure good fetal evolution

Giving you time to watch and wait

And allow delivery at a later date.

With abruptions of grade 2

There is basically one thing to do

And that, Metzler, will let you know

Is get to the OR. Go! Go! Go!

The bleeding is much greater, hence

The uterus feels tender and tense.

With pain not resolving between contractions

The outcome depends on your reactions.

The monitor shows fetal distress

If you don't deliver Grade 2 will progress

Like an avalanche, into Grade 3

So, quickly now, start your IV's

Draw your labs, your type and cross

Do a Cesarean. You must be the boss

And direct the crew in this situation.

Especially when there is hesitation.

With Grade 2 abruption, the baby you might save

But in Grade 3, alas, it is the grave

Ultimately, that awaits this tiny creature,

And to avoid a double feature,

Mom and babe, time do not neglect

Hypovolemic shock you must correct.

You will start by giving crystalloid

But blood products you won't avoid.

Coagulopathy you need to correct.

In doing this you must inspect

The H/H, platelet count and fibrinogen

To give you an idea where to begin.

In addition to red blood cell transfusions

You need FFP and platelet infusions

And sometimes cryoprecipitate

All must be considered, before it's too late.

And the mother goes into DIC

Or has a consumptive coagulopathy.

And despite your heroic surgery

She joins the baby in the mortuary.

So keep a high index of suspicion

And don't be plagued by indecision.

Shoulder Dystocia

It's the moment that we all dread

You've just delivered the baby's head.

But when you try to deliver the shoulder

It feels like trying to move a boulder.

And in this moment of despair

As you offer a silent prayer

You'll ask yourself how one so fertile

Can have the head scrunched like a turtle.

Before we go forward, lets look back

To see what caused your anxiety attack.

It seems now just a little late

To estimate the fetal weight.

Did you forget to eat your Wheaties?

Did the Mom have diabetes?

Is the patient short and stout?

Unable to push the baby out?

Perhaps it was that vacuum cup

That got you stuck in all this muck.

If not the vacuum, maybe blades

Caused this awful escapade.

Epidural motor block?

Let's get going, we're on the clock.

Deisher's voice I'd hear inflect

Should one go pulling on the neck.

Because it is the baby's arm

Ultimately one will harm

By this strong but foolish action.

Do not engage cervical traction!

Erb-Duchenne and Klumpke palsies

Will result, and if we cause these

The arm will hang like some pip,

Of a waiter asking for a tip.

The cervical nerves five through eight

Can be injured, so hesitate.

Lest you meet Duncan, Bickel and Burn

Or some other plaintiffs lawyer firm

Who will ask during your deposition

What other maneuvers or position

You tried before stretching out the neck

And the nerves of the brachial plexus did wreck

Episiotomy? There's a debate

As to whether this will help create

More room to let the shoulders slip through.

Episiotomy? Some don't and some do.

But, don't lose hope, there is a way

To deliver the shoulders and save the day

First off, do like McRoberts said

And position the patient on the bed

Like a cheerleader awaiting the reception

Of the star quarterback's impending conception

Ankles thrown back to the ears

This will help the shoulder clear

Underneath the symphysis pubis

This is the first step in the rubric

If this maneuver doesn't work

Do not pull harder or try to jerk

Instead, one rotates the posterior shoulder

With two fingers near the axillary fold there

Push around towards the back

Wood's screw it's called, to get the knack

Practice when doing deliveries routine

Most of the time, it works like a dream.

(Also tried as a measure

Is giving suprapubic pressure

My experience, I must confess

Is this rarely helps resolve the mess.)

When Wood's and old McRobert's fail

Do not panic, one can prevail

With a trick that takes a lot of sand:

Reaching up for the baby's hand

This takes quite a bit of strength

Fingers strong and good in length

One makes the hand into a wedge

And forces it past the baby's head

Along the anterior of the chest

Reaching up 'til it comes to rest

With the babies hand in one's grasp

Then, pulling down, one sweeps it past

The chest and head, works like a charm

Its how one delivers the posterior arm.

For shoulder dystocia so severe

The head won't come out past the ear

There is the famous Zavanelli

Push the head back in the belly

To the OR lickety-split.

Do a Cesarean. Quickly. Do it.

Afterwards, you might tell the tale

"A baby sized much like a whale."

'Tis sadly the case that braggadocio

Accompanies stories of dystocia.

Premature Rupture of Membranes

When a patient calls, these words are often spoken:

"Doc, I hate to tell you, I think my water's broken.

I just went to the bathroom and right after the flush

I stood up by the toilet and I felt a sudden gush."

Now, as the patient's standing, the head drops on the bladder

This causes her to urinate, that's usually what's the matter.

But, diagnostic telephone will get you into trouble.

So have the patient come right in, and tell her "on the double."

At times the diagnosis, is quite simple to make

A glance at the vagina is really all it takes.

But when there's not gross rupture, sometimes it isn't clear.

The labor nurse informs you, "There's no fluid down there.

I checked this gal with Nitrazine and it didn't turn blue.

I don't think that she's ruptured. What do you want to do?"

You answer very gently, "Thank you much good Ma'am.

But I need to be thorough, do a speculum exam."

So you look at the cervix, take a little peak

Everything is dry there, not even a wee leak.

But Nitrazine is positive, yet, you don't see any fern

But wait, what's that there swimming; it's a tiny little sperm.

And another, and another, makes the diagnosis simple

Her water isn't broken; she's been with old Dalrymple.

Still other times despite all tests, rupture is equivocal

One can't conclude things either way, so you're perplexed and quizzical

Roll around the ultrasound, check the uterus for fluid.

Taking still another step, inject indigo carmine into it.

The diagnosis of P-ROM will then be clear to you

If after walking 'round a bit, the patient's leaking blue.

This isn't needed nowadays, intactness you ensure

By doing now a new test, one called Amnisure.

This placental amnioglobulin, immunoassay test

Can answer all your questions and put ROM to rest.

Heed me now, the *Rule of Finger*

Never let your digits linger

In the cervix when the water breaks

Because that is all that it takes

To start infection's ticking clock

Keep your fingers on the dock

And use speculum instead.

Don't use your fingers, use your head.

How we manage PROM, according to the sages

Is pretty much determined by the gestational ages.

Balancing infection versus prematurity

One must pick their poison. Oh what insecurity!

For patients who present at 34 weeks or greater

It's best to move toward delivery, sooner rather than later.

But, if the pregnancy, in weeks is dated less

To expectant management we're forced to acquiesce.

So we give our steroids to help the lungs mature.

Watch closely for infections- the signs can be obscure.

If on ultrasound there's a pocket that is clear

Amniocentesis, can provide good info here.

Be on the lookout, for signs of an abruption

Cord prolapse too might cause some sleep disruption.

Especially in those cases when the feet are coming first

You hang out in the call room, hoping you're not cursed.

Finally, the last thing that I want to teach

Is what to do when viability is out of reach.

Such as when there's P-ROM, at only 16 weeks

Alas, the saddened patient, a miracle she seeks.

With oligohydramnios, she hasn't got a prayer

And to give her false hope, well is it really fair?

Exposing her to sepsis, for such little gain

From this type of management I think we should refrain.

Giving her autonomy doesn't mean we should

Speak to her of options, which aren't any good.

The End

www.ingramcontent.com/pod-product-compliance
Lightning Source LLC
Chambersburg PA
CBHW021415170526
45164CB00002B/662